Dyslexic Sup

Techniques for Succeeding: Unleashing Your Potential to Turn Reading Difficulties into Creative Chances in Education, Employment, and Life

Michele L. Valdez

Introducing the exclusive and captivating world of Michele L. Valdez. Immerse yourself in the timeless elegance and creativity that defines our brand. Experience the unparalleled craftsmanship and attention to detail that sets us apart. Discover the essence of sophistication and style with our exquisite collection. Copyright © 2024 Michele L. Valdez

Table of Contents

P r e f a c e

Are you prepared to tap into your unlimited potential and fully embrace your unique brilliance as a dyslexic individual? Step into a world of empowerment, inspiration, and transformation. Within the pages of our upcoming book, " Dyslexic Superpowers: Harnessing Your Unique Powers," you will embark on a transformative journey that is truly unparalleled.

In a society that frequently emphasizes constraints, we aim to redefine the perception of dyslexia. Dyslexia will no longer be viewed as an obstacle to achievement, but rather as a route to extraordinary accomplishments. Our book goes beyond mere comprehension of dyslexia; it encourages acceptance, appreciation, and tapping into its remarkable capabilities.

Celebrating Your Uniqueness

We begin your journey by embracing and honoring the distinctiveness of dyslexia. Creative thinking and problem-solving skills are just a few of the many advantages that dyslexia brings, which are often overlooked by traditional education systems. With captivating narratives and thought-provoking examples, you'll gain a fresh perspective on dyslexia.

Unleashing Your Hidden Talents

Prepare to explore the depths of your dyslexic abilities. Discover the exceptional talents that distinguish you, whether it's your innovative thinking, ability to grasp intricate ideas, or knack for making insightful connections. With hands-on activities and the guidance of experienced professionals, you will discover how to utilize these abilities to make your dreams a reality.

Embracing Difficulties with Assurance

We acknowledge the difficulties that accompany living with dyslexia. Rest assured, we are here to provide you with the necessary tools and strategies to conquer any challenge. By honing your time management skills and overcoming self-doubt, you will develop a newfound strength and resilience that will empower you to confidently face any challenge that comes your way.

Succeeding in Academia and Beyond Education is merely the starting point of your adventure. Whether you're a student navigating the intricacies of the classroom or a professional striving for success in the workplace, our book will guide you on how to excel in any setting. By providing practical tips, proven techniques, and real-world advice, this resource will guide you in transforming your dyslexia into a valuable asset.

Creating a Supportive Community

It's important that nobody has to face this journey by themselves. That's why we stress the significance of creating a nurturing community of supporters, guides, and others who share the experience of dyslexia. Whether you're browsing through online forums or attending local meetups, you'll find a plethora of valuable resources and valuable connections to support you on your journey.

Embracing Your Future with Assurance

As you approach the concluding chapters of our book, you will experience a surge of motivation and a world of new opportunities opening up before you. With a deep understanding of your unique strengths and abilities, you will fearlessly forge ahead, poised to leave a lasting impact on the world.

This is only the beginning of your journey; it doesn't end here. When you have "Unleashing Dyslexic Brilliance" as your guide, the possibilities become limitless. So why hesitate any longer? Embark on an extraordinary journey and unlock your limitless potential now!

Get your hands on it before anyone else!

Experience the incredible opportunity to be one of the pioneers on this life-changing adventure. Secure your pre-order of "Unleashing Dyslexic Brilliance" now and enjoy a range of exclusive bonuses. Gain entry to our vibrant online community, delve into bonus chapters, and gain behind-the-scenes insights. Don't pass up this chance to uncover your extraordinary abilities and transform your life indefinitely.

Testimonials: *"This book has completely transformed my understanding of dyslexia. I used to view it as a chore, but now I perceive it as a blessing. Thank you for enlightening me! -* **Sarah H., person with dyslexia**

"This book has made a significant impact on my life as a parent of a dyslexic child. It has equipped me with the necessary resources and self-assurance to guide my child towards a path of achievement." - **John D., concerned parent**

"I really could have used this book during my childhood." It would have spared me countless years of hardship and uncertainty. Thank you for providing such a valuable resource. - **Emily S., adult with dyslexia**

Be a part of the Movement

Working together, we have the power to reshape the perception of dyslexia and inspire countless individuals worldwide. Join us today and become a part of an exceptional movement. Tap into your unique perspective and make a lasting impact - one page at a time.

Introduction

Are you exhausted from the constant frustration of dyslexia hindering your progress? In "Dyslexic Superpowers," the esteemed author, Michele L. Valdez presents a groundbreaking investigation into the unexplored capabilities of individuals with dyslexia. This book will completely transform your understanding of dyslexia with its captivating narratives, effective techniques, and valuable perspectives from professionals.

Michele L. Valdez, reveals the fascinating reality of dyslexia. It goes beyond being a mere learning difference; it is actually an untapped superpower. With captivating real-life stories and groundbreaking research, Michele L. Valdez challenges the common misconceptions about dyslexia and sheds light on the remarkable abilities it grants to individuals.

Uncover the exceptional abilities that dyslexia brings, including a boost in creativity and problem-solving abilities, as well as a heightened sense of empathy and spatial awareness. Through practical techniques and empowering activities, this book leads readers on a life-changing path to fully embrace their dyslexic identity and harness its power for extraordinary achievements in all areas of life.

Whether you're a parent looking to support your child's growth, an educator working towards inclusive learning environments, or an adult navigating the professional world, Dyslexic Superpowers provides valuable insights and practical tools to unleash the full potential of dyslexia.

Celebrate your unique qualities. Tap into your extraordinary abilities. Transform your life with Dyslexic Superpowers.

Uncover the Distinctive Benefits:

- Embrace dyslexia as a unique strength, rather than a hindrance

- Unleash your boundless creativity and innovation like never before

- Tap into the potential of thinking outside the box to tackle intricate challenges

- Achieve success in academia, career, and personal pursuits

Inspiring Stories: From conquering challenges to reaching extraordinary heights, "Dyslexic Superpowers" presents compelling stories of individuals with dyslexia who have surpassed expectations and embraced their exceptional talents. No matter if you're a parent, educator, or someone who has dyslexia, this book will motivate and empower you to fully embrace dyslexia with confidence and pride.

Useful Resources and Techniques:

Filled with practical advice and effective strategies, "Dyslexic Superpowers" provides you with the resources necessary to thrive in a world that favors neurotypical individuals. This book provides practical solutions for overcoming the challenges of dyslexia and excelling in all areas of life, including improving reading comprehension, memory, and concentration.

Get on board with the revolution:

It's high time we break down the barriers associated with dyslexia and unleash the untapped potential of dyslexic individuals across the globe. Become part of the movement and fully embrace the incredible strengths of dyslexia today!

Celebrate your unique qualities. Tap into your extraordinary abilities. Transform your life with Dyslexic Superpowers.

Chapter 1

Discover the Fascinating World of Dyslexia

Discover the challenges faced by individuals with dyslexia as they navigate the world of reading and writing.

- Discover the fascinating truth: cleverness and dyslexia are not linked.

- Discover the power of early diagnosis, expert guidance, and unwavering support to minimize the impact of dyslexia.

- Introducing a groundbreaking discovery: individuals with dyslexia may experience a range of immunological challenges.

Discover the fascinating world of Dyslexia!

Experience the challenges of dyslexia as it impacts word recognition, spelling, and decoding abilities.

Unlock the hidden potential within individuals with dyslexia as their minds embark on a unique journey of processing written materials. Discover the ultimate solution to effortlessly identify, spell, and decipher words with absolute ease.

Discover the challenges faced by individuals with dyslexia as they navigate the world of reading. Discover the fascinating world of dyslexia, a remarkable neurological condition that can sometimes have a genetic component. Unlike popular misconceptions, dyslexia is not caused by inadequate teaching, training, or upbringing. It's a unique trait that sets individuals apart.

Discover the astonishing fact that between five and fifteen percent of individuals in the United States are affected by dyslexia.

Discover the Truth: Diagnosis

Discover the key to unlocking your child's potential. If you suspect that your little one may have dyslexia, don't wait another moment. Take action now and reach out to the experts at your child's school for a professional evaluation. Together, we can pave the way for a brighter future. Discover the power of early analysis, which greatly increases the chances of achieving effective treatment.

Discover the endless possibilities that test results can unlock for your child. By obtaining these results, your child may gain access to a world of support, including special education services, tailored support programs, and a wide range of services offered by prestigious universities and colleges.

Discover the wide range of areas that diagnostic tests can cover:

- Discover the power of background information and the art of intelligence.

- Enhance your dental language skills.

- Introducing the incredible power of word recognition.

- Unlock the power of decoding, the key to effortlessly reading new words by harnessing the incredible potential of letter-sound knowledge.

- Experience the power of phonological processing.

- Enhance your automaticity and fluency skills with our cutting-edge program.

- Enhance your reading comprehension and expand your vocabulary knowledge.

- Uncover the fascinating world of genealogy and delve into the intriguing early development of this captivating field.

Unlock the power of the assessment process as our skilled examiner expertly navigates through a myriad of possibilities, eliminating any other conditions or factors that may masquerade as similar symptoms. Trust in their expertise to uncover the truth. Introducing a range of challenges that can impact our daily lives, such as eyesight problems, hearing impairment, insufficient instruction, as well as sociable and financial factors.

Experience the telltale signs

Discover the fascinating world of dyslexia, a unique condition that sets it apart from mere delayed reading development. Unlike other factors such as mental impairment or cultural deprivation, dyslexia presents a distinct set of challenges and opportunities.

Discover the telltale signs of dyslexia that can manifest at any age, but are most commonly observed during childhood.

Discover the telltale signs of dyslexia in children, including the common struggle of deciphering the written word.

Discover the remarkable potential of children with dyslexia. Despite their normal intelligence and receiving the best teaching and parental support, they face the challenge of unlocking the world of reading.

Experience the thrill of reaching milestones later than ever before!

Discover the incredible journey of children with dyslexia as they conquer milestones like crawling, walking, chatting, and even riding a bike, albeit at their own unique pace.

Experience the wonder of delayed speech development.

Introducing the remarkable journey of a young individual with dyslexia. Witness their determination as they navigate the intricacies of speech, overcoming obstacles that others may take for granted. With unwavering perseverance, they conquer the art of pronunciation, unravel the mysteries of rhyming, and embark on a quest to distinguish between the subtle nuances of various word sounds.

Discover the power of reducing learning units of data!

Discover the incredible journey of college students with dyslexia as they navigate the fascinating world of language. Witness their determination as they conquer the challenge of understanding the intricate characters of the alphabet and unravel the secrets of pronunciation. Experience the triumph of knowledge and the power of perseverance. Introducing the ultimate solution for keeping track of the ever-changing times of the week, the four seasons, a plethora of vibrant colors, and even those pesky arithmetic tables. Say goodbye to forgetfulness and hello to seamless organization with our revolutionary system.

Introducing: Coordination Discover how your child can overcome clumsiness and stand out from their peers. Experience the thrill of acquiring a ball like never before! Discover the fascinating connection between eye-hand coordination and neurological conditions like dyspraxia. Uncover the hidden indicators that could shed light on a deeper understanding of these conditions.

Unraveling the Enigma: Discovering the Root Causes of Dyslexia

Discover the truth about dyslexia - it's not an illness, but rather a unique challenge that can occur within families from birth. Discover the truth about individuals with dyslexia - they are anything but ridiculous or sluggish. Unlock the potential of your mind with our extraordinary individuals who possess exceptional cleverness. Witness their relentless dedication as they conquer any learning obstacles that come their way.

Discover the fascinating world of dyslexia, where groundbreaking research reveals that this condition is intricately linked to the way our brains process information. Behold the captivating imagery of the mind, revealing a fascinating truth: those with dyslexia possess a unique cognitive landscape when it comes to reading. Unlike their non-dyslexic counterparts, they engage diverse regions of the mind in this intricate process. Behold, these captivating pictures serve as undeniable proof that the intricate workings of the human brain, when afflicted by dyslexia, fail to function optimally when engaged in the noble act of reading. Discover the secret to effortless reading and unlock a world of knowledge.

Discover the impact of Dyslexia on your life.

Discover the fascinating truth about dyslexia, a condition that captivates the minds of many. Contrary to popular belief, dyslexia doesn't simply cause letters and figures to change, or words to be read backwards. Let's delve deeper into the intricacies of this intriguing phenomenon. Experience the natural ebb and flow of growth with the occasional twist and turn. Reversals are a common occurrence that many children encounter during their early stages of development.

Discover the key challenge in dyslexia: difficulty in recognizing phonemes. Introducing the fundamental essence of conversation, phonemes like the "b" audio in "bat" hold the power to captivate. They present a unique challenge, as they seamlessly merge with the fabric of speech, making it difficult to visually grasp their symbolic representation and effortlessly blend them into words.

Experience the challenge of identifying concise, well-known words or deciphering complex, lengthier words. Unlock the potential of individuals with dyslexia by providing them with the time and focus they need to decode words. Word reading may require extra effort, but with patience and practice, they can overcome any challenge. Discover the world through the eyes of someone with dyslexia, where every word becomes a captivating maze and comprehension feels like an elusive treasure.

Discover the unsurprising fact that individuals with dyslexia often encounter challenges when it comes to spelling. Moreover, they might encounter difficulty articulating their thoughts both in written form and in verbal communication. Introducing Dyslexia: The Ultimate Vocabulary Processing Disorder

Discover the fascinating world of dyslexia, where many individuals experience milder forms of this condition. These individuals may find themselves navigating the realms of spoken and written vocabulary with greater ease. Discover how countless individuals overcome the challenges of dyslexia with unwavering determination and an unwavering commitment to go the extra mile. Discover the truth about dyslexia - a condition that doesn't simply vanish or fade away with time. Discover the incredible power of proper assistance, enabling countless individuals with dyslexia to unlock the ability to read. Discover the myriad of ways they frequently employ to comprehend and effectively utilize those strategies in their everyday lives.

Discover the challenges of dyslexia, where even the most familiar words can become a daunting task to read. Prepare to embark on a journey of gradual reading, where you'll find yourself compelled to push your limits and work diligently to absorb every word. Discover the art of letter mixing in a nutshell. Imagine the thrill of reading the word "now" and experiencing the sensation of "received". Or how about encountering the word "left" and being transported to the realm of "experienced"? Unleash your imagination and embrace the power of letter play. Experience the seamless harmony of words effortlessly blending together, where every space is filled with purpose and nothing is lost.

Introducing the ultimate solution for those who struggle with remembering what they've read. Experience the power of personalized learning and auditory stimulation.

Enhance your memory retention by having information read to you or listening to it. Discover the effortless way to remember with ease. Unlock the secrets of mathematical problem-solving with our expert guidance. Tackle even the toughest phrase problems with confidence, showcasing your mastery of arithmetic fundamentals. Let us empower you to conquer the challenges that lie ahead.

Are you struggling to find the perfect words or names for the various objects during your pre-class demonstration? Look no further! Discover the challenges that individuals with dyslexia face when it comes to spelling and writing.

Discover the process of diagnosing Dyslexia.

Discover the ingenious ways that individuals with dyslexia overcome their challenges, skillfully concealing any signs of difficulty. Discover the secret to avoiding embarrassment and unlocking a world of ease in school and reading: seeking help. Say goodbye to struggles and hello to success with a little assistance. Discover the remarkable journey of individuals who are diagnosed at a young age, but brace yourself for the surprising truth - it's not uncommon for teenagers and even adults to receive their diagnosis.

Discover the telltale signs of dyslexia that parents and educators should be on the lookout for:

Discover the untapped potential within, even with normal intelligence. Unlock the power of effective communication with enhanced reading, spelling, and writing skills.

Are you constantly struggling to complete projects and meet deadlines? We understand the frustration that comes with not being able to finish tasks on time. Let us help you overcome this challenge and ensure that you never miss another deadline again.

Struggling to recall the right brands for various products?

Experience the frustration of struggling to remember written lists and telephone numbers? Say goodbye to that struggle with our revolutionary memory-boosting solution. Unlock your brain's full potential and never forget important information again.

Are you tired of struggling with directions and reading maps? Say goodbye to the confusion of figuring out which way is up or down. Let us help you navigate with ease and confidence.

Experience a seamless journey through your classes with our innovative solutions.

Discovering that you have any of these problems does not necessarily mean that you have dyslexia. But someone who shows several indications ought to be examined for the problem.

Experience a comprehensive physical examination that includes thorough hearing and eyesight evaluations, expertly designed to identify and address any potential medical concerns. Discover the true potential of your language, reading, spelling, and writing abilities with a comprehensive array of standardized tests administered by a highly skilled college psychologist or learning specialist. Unlock the power of your mind with an extraordinary test of thinking ability - the IQ test. Challenge yourself and discover your true intellectual potential. Discover the challenges that individuals with dyslexia often face in various academic areas, such as handwriting and mathematics. Additionally, they may encounter difficulties with focus and memory. In such instances, alternative testing methods can be explored to ensure accurate assessment.

Discover Effective Strategies for Thriving with Dyslexia

Discover how to overcome the challenges of dyslexia with the assistance that's readily accessible. Discover the power of inclusive education! According to the latest legislation, individuals diagnosed with a learning impairment, such as dyslexia, are entitled to receive exceptional support from all members of the school community. Unlock their full potential with our comprehensive assistance program. Unlock the potential of young minds with dyslexia through the guidance of a specially trained teacher, tutor, or reading specialist. Watch as they embark on a transformative journey to master the art of reading and spelling with confidence.

Discover the ultimate form of assistance that imparts the invaluable knowledge of speech sounds in words, also known as phonemic awareness, and the magical connection between letters and sounds, commonly referred to as phonics. Discover the power of tailored learning and practice activities designed specifically for students with dyslexia. Unlock their true potential with the guidance of a skilled instructor or teacher.

Unlocking the full potential of students with dyslexia is a top priority. That's why we provide them with invaluable resources to ensure their success. From granting them extra time to complete projects or tests, to allowing them to record class lectures, or even providing copies of lecture notes - we go above and beyond to empower these students to thrive. Enhance your written assignments with the help of a computer equipped with advanced spelling checkers. Experience the convenience and accuracy that comes with this innovative tool. Introducing an exceptional solution for older students in demanding classes - a range of services that go above and beyond. Imagine having access to recorded versions of any book, yes, even textbooks! Elevate your learning experience like never before. Discover the incredible world of applications that have the power to "read" printed material aloud! Unlock the potential of this amazing technology by simply reaching out to your parent, teacher, or learning disability services coordinator. They will guide you on the exciting journey of accessing these remarkable services. Don't miss out on this opportunity to enhance your learning experience!

Experience the power of emotional support. Discover the struggle of individuals with dyslexia, who tirelessly strive to keep up with their peers, only to be left frustrated and disheartened. Discover the hidden brilliance within them. Sometimes, they may mistakenly believe that their intelligence pales in comparison to their peers. But fear not, for they have a clever way of masking their insecurities. They may choose to dazzle their classmates with their antics or assume the role of the class clown. Experience the power of collaboration as they strive to attract more students to join them in achieving their goals. Discover the art of pretending, where the true value of grades becomes a mere illusion and the notion of school being dumb is playfully contemplated.

Discover the incredible power of support from family and friends in assisting individuals with dyslexia. It's crucial to recognize that these individuals are not unintelligent or unmotivated. By encouraging them to give their best effort, we can unlock their true potential. Discover and celebrate the unique talents of every individual, whether they excel in sports, performing arts, visual arts, innovative thinking, or any other remarkable pursuit.

Unlock your true potential and rise above the challenges of dyslexia. Don't let it hold you back in your academic pursuits or career aspirations. Embrace your unique strengths and conquer any obstacles that come your way. Discover how colleges go above and beyond to support students with dyslexia. Experience the advantage of trained tutors, cutting-edge learning aids, innovative applications, convenient recorded reading assignments, and personalized exam arrangements. Embrace a learning environment that caters to your unique needs.

Unlocking the potential within, individuals with dyslexia have the power to soar to great heights. With their unique perspective and unwavering determination, they can conquer any field they choose. From the noble profession of medicine to the captivating world of politics, from the dynamic realm of corporate leadership to the enchanting realm of the arts, the possibilities are limitless. They can grace the silver screen as talented actors, captivate audiences with their melodious tunes as gifted musicians, create awe-inspiring masterpieces as visionary artists, impart knowledge and shape young minds as dedicated teachers, revolutionize industries as ingenious inventors, and even pave their own path as fearless entrepreneurs. The world is their canvas, and they have the power to paint it with their extraordinary talents. Discover the awe-inspiring journeys of numerous dyslexic celebrities who have triumphed over reading challenges to achieve remarkable success in their respective fields and beyond.

Discover the Path to Overcoming

Dyslexia!

Absolutely not. Discover the enduring impact of dyslexia, a lifelong condition that accompanies individuals throughout their journey into old age. Discover the incredible power of education to transform the lives of individuals with dyslexia and unlock their full potential in written vocabulary. Discover the wealth of evidence that reveals the specific types of training that struggling readers require to achieve success. Esteemed sources such as the Countrywide Institute of Child Medical health insurance and Person Development (2000), Snow et al. (1998), and Torgesen (2000) have all contributed to this body of knowledge.

Introducing a groundbreaking study that delves into the fascinating world of children's minds! Prepare to be amazed as our team of analysts explores the impact of a rigorous intervention on the brain activity of children with RD. For the first time ever, we will uncover the hidden consequences and shed light on the remarkable changes that take place. Brace yourself for a mind-blowing journey!

Introducing to you, not one, but two remarkable studies that are sure to captivate your attention.

Witness the groundbreaking study conducted by Aylward et al. (2003), where the minds of ten remarkable children with dyslexia were meticulously examined. Not stopping there, the study also included eleven individuals of average abilities for a comprehensive comparison. Brace yourself for the astonishing results that unfolded after a transformative twenty-eight-hour treatment, exclusively administered to the dyslexic students. Prepare to be amazed! Discover the remarkable similarities between both groups of students when it comes to their performance on out-of-magnet reading assessments and the level of engagement they exhibit while identifying notice sounds.

Discover the fascinating results of their study! While the control children failed to demonstrate any notable differences between the two imaging methods, the students who were given the task experienced a remarkable surge in activation. This increase occurred specifically in the areas crucial for reading and language, all thanks to the phonological task they undertook. Witness the remarkable transformation of these young individuals with RD. Prior to the intervention, their potential was hindered by significant under-activation in crucial areas, setting them apart from their peers. However, with the power of effective treatment, their profiles underwent a stunning metamorphosis, becoming virtually indistinguishable from those of the control children. Prepare to be amazed by the incredible results!

Discover the intriguing results that await, but proceed with caution as we navigate the realm of limitations. Introducing a few limitations that may arise: first, there is often a lack of specificity regarding the provided participation. Additionally, the test size tends to be on the smaller side, which can impact the results. Lastly, there is a lack of an experimental control group, meaning that many children with RD did not undergo the procedure. These limitations should be taken into consideration. Without the presence of an experimental control group, it is impossible to guarantee that the procedure alone was responsible for the changes in mind activation. Numerous other potential explanations could have influenced the results.

Discover how Shaywitz et al. (2004) brilliantly tackled the limitations by conducting a groundbreaking analysis of the fascinating changes in brain activation before and after engagement. Introducing a groundbreaking study that delved into the lives of not just any students, but seventy-eight exceptional second and third graders with reading disabilities. These remarkable individuals were carefully selected and randomly assigned to one of three distinguished groups, each with its own unique purpose and potential for growth:

- The experimental intervention group, where innovative strategies and techniques were employed to unlock their true reading potential.

- The school-based remedial programs group, where tried-and-true methods were utilized to provide targeted support and guidance.

- And lastly, the Control group, which served as the benchmark against which the other groups were measured. Prepare to be amazed as we unveil the fascinating findings of this extraordinary study!

Chapter 2

Discover the groundbreaking world of intervention in brain imaging research for dyslexic children.

Experience the power of our personalized tutoring intervention program. With sessions that take place day-by-day for a total of fifty minutes, from September to June, we ensure consistent and effective support for every student. Our program boasts an impressive average of one hundred and twenty-six sessions or a hundred and five tutoring hours per student. Trust us to help your child reach their full potential.

Introducing: The Ultimate Guide to Mastering Your Skills!

Experience the power of our tutoring sessions, meticulously designed to provide a framework of five essential steps that our dedicated tutors follow with each and every student. Unlock your full potential with our proven approach. Introducing a groundbreaking platform that goes beyond scripted lessons. Our platform is uniquely tailored to each student's progress, ensuring a truly personalized learning experience.

Discover the fascinating world of sound-symbol human relationships in a concise and fast-paced summary of previous lessons. Get ready to dive into exciting new correspondences that will expand your knowledge even further.

Experience the transformative power of phonemic segmentation and blending with our innovative letter charge cards or tiles. Our method is meticulously designed to ensure a systematic and explicit approach, guaranteeing optimal results.

Enhance your fluency with a captivating array of words and phonetically regular words carefully crafted using sound-symbol correspondences you've already learned.

Experience the joy of dental reading practice with our phonetically managed text, uncontrolled trade books, and captivating non-fiction texts. Enhance your skills and immerse yourself in a world of knowledge and entertainment. Start your journey today!

Experience the power of writing words with previously taught patterns from dictation. Unlock your potential and enhance your language skills with this transformative exercise. Embrace the art of spelling and watch as your vocabulary expands before your very eyes. Step into a world of linguistic mastery and let your words flow effortlessly onto the page. Prepare to be amazed as you witness the magic of dictation unfold.

Experience the power of our intervention program, designed to take you on a journey through six levels of language mastery. Begin with the elegance of simple closed syllable words like "kitty," and watch as your skills grow, culminating in the triumph of conquering multisyllabic words that encompass all six syllable types. Unleash your linguistic potential today!

Witness the remarkable transformation that occurred after the intervention. Initially, all groups displayed comparable levels of brain activity. However, in a stunning turn of events, both the experimental and control groups experienced a surge in activation within the hemispheric regions that are absolutely vital for reading. Prepare to be amazed by the power of this intervention!

Experience the remarkable results of our intervention program! Just one year later, the experimental group demonstrated a significant boost in activity within the occipito-temporal region. This enhanced activation is essential for achieving automated, fluent reading. What's more, our program also led to a reduction in compensatory activation in the correct hemisphere over time. Witness the power of our cutting-edge approach!

Discover the groundbreaking findings of Shaywitz et al. (2002) as they unveil the remarkable benefits of incorporating the evidence-based phonologic reading treatment. Their conclusive results shed light on the incredible impact this treatment has on the development of the fast-paced neural systems that are the foundation of skilled reading. Prepare to be amazed by the transformative power of this cutting-edge approach!

Discover the Crucial Factors to Observe Regarding Brain Research

Introducing groundbreaking research advancements that grant us an unprecedented glimpse into the inner workings of your brain, unveiling crucial insights into the intricacies of our thoughts while engaged in reading. However, it is imperative to bear in mind certain essential considerations that demand our attention.

Introducing the groundbreaking report by the esteemed B.E. Shaywitz, S. Shaywitz, and their esteemed team of co-workers. Prepare to be amazed as we delve into the world of research, where the test sizes in each study are nothing short of remarkable. Discover the power of knowledge as these small studies converge into reliable results. Keep in mind, the findings may evolve as more individuals join the study foundation. Discover the undeniable truth about children's education, where both the level of academic achievement and the size of tests have significantly diminished.

Introducing the second crucial factor to ponder: the

nature of the task performed within the magnetic realm. Discover the fascinating world of brain imaging research! Unfortunately, due to certain limitations, researchers are unable to study individuals while they are reading aloud. But fear not, there are still countless other exciting avenues to explore in the realm of neuroscience! Introducing a revolutionary approach, they offer captivating tasks that encourage individuals to embark on a journey of silent learning. With a simple push of a button, one can effortlessly determine if the characters 't' and 'v' create a harmonious rhyme. Discover the mesmerizing world of rhyme! Have you ever wondered if "leat" and "jete" dance to the same beat? Let's unravel this poetic mystery together.

Introducing a team of meticulously selected professionals who have diligently worked on these tasks, ensuring a system that is both precise and reliable. Rest assured, their expert analysis of the activation amounts can be trusted. However, it is important to note that the nature of these tasks has deviated from the conventional reading, making direct comparisons somewhat challenging.

Experience the rapid advancement of brain research as it pushes the boundaries of scientific exploration. Witness the remarkable technological breakthroughs that hold the promise of resolving these challenges in the near future.

Discover the Ultimate Selection of Options for Teachers!

Discover the profound implications of this wealth of information for college staff and their students. Discover the essential processes and key factors behind reading disabilities, empowering educators to harness this knowledge and forge meaningful connections with their students and themselves. Discover the power of these meticulously crafted suggestions, carefully derived from cutting-edge neurological research:

Discover the crucial importance of conducting a thorough assessment of language processing when it comes to understanding the root causes behind students' struggles in learning how to regulate their learning effectively.

Introducing Dyslexia, the reading impairment that challenges the very core of your brain's vocabulary control systems. Discover the precise types of weaknesses that can be found and unlock the key to finding the perfect teaching method tailored to meet each student's unique needs.

Discover the groundbreaking findings of imaging research, which unequivocally establish that seemingly effortless tasks may indeed serve as unmistakable "warning flags," indicating a potential risk for dyslexia in children.

Unlock the potential of young minds by implementing cutting-edge testing and improvement monitoring procedures right from the start. Measure children's knowledge of sound in speech, observe their ability to identify sounds in words, and enhance their fluency in word recognition. Discover the power of ongoing evaluation in a child's educational journey. By utilizing this effective tool, teachers gain valuable insights into which skills to focus on and can track a child's progress. Stay ahead of the game and ensure that your child is developing the necessary skills for success.

Discover the transformative power of explicit, intense,

and systematic instructions in the audio structure of vocabulary (phonemic recognition) and the seamless connection between sounds and words (phonics). These invaluable techniques are essential for individuals with dyslexia, unlocking their full potential and paving the way for success.

Discover the groundbreaking findings of imaging research that has unequivocally confirmed the profound impact of instruction in the alphabetic principle. Prepare to be amazed as you learn about the distinct variations in brain activation patterns that have been observed in students with RD. Brace yourself for a paradigm-shifting revelation that will revolutionize the way we approach education. (Shaywitz et al., 2004) Discover the profound nature of the task at hand - one that is explicit, extreme, and long-term. This task is specifically centered around the art of phonological handling, phonics, and fluency. Embrace the challenge and dive into the world of language mastery.

Discover the indispensable roles of motivation and the fear of failure when delving into the realm of reading problems.

Unlock your full potential as a student and leave behind the days of struggling. It's not about trying harder, it's about discovering the right approach to success. Discover the fascinating world of individuals who possess a unique brain difference, which allows them to perceive and comprehend the world around them in a remarkably profound manner, surpassing that of their peers. Experience the transformative power of our cutting-edge intervention techniques to prevent the development of low inspiration in students. Say goodbye to avoiding hard and painful tasks and unlock your true potential.

Discover the power of leveraging neurological characteristics and the basis of dyslexia to empower students in their journey of understanding reading and vocabulary. School personnel are equipped with the knowledge to help students embrace their unique strengths and weaknesses.

Discover the key to unraveling the enigma and overcoming the challenges that many individuals with disabilities face. By understanding the underlying reasons behind their unique struggles, they can unlock the door to learning difficult concepts that seem to baffle others. This newfound knowledge will not only assist them in their journey but also alleviate the mystery and negative emotions associated with their disability. Unlock the secrets of brain research and unravel the mysteries of dyslexia. By shedding light on this fascinating subject, we can empower students and their parents to see that vocabulary processing is not a daunting challenge, but rather one of the many unique talents they possess. Let's dispel the notion of being "ridiculous" and instead celebrate the diverse ways in which they process language.

Chapter 3

Discover the fascinating world of Brain Imaging!

Unlock the secrets of the mind with a myriad of cutting-edge techniques designed to visualize the intricate world of brain anatomy and function. Introducing the remarkable Magnetic Resonance Imaging (MRI) - the ultimate tool you can trust. With its unparalleled ability to create stunning images, MRI unveils a wealth of information about brain anatomy. Discover the intricate details of grey and white matter, and witness the pristine integrity of white matter. But that's not all - MRI goes beyond the surface, delving into the realm of brain metabolites. Explore the fascinating world of chemicals that facilitate communication between brain cells. And let's not forget about brain function - MRI takes you on a journey to witness the vibrant energy of large pools of neurons. Brace yourself for a mind-blowing experience with MRI! Introducing the groundbreaking technology of Functional MRI (fMRI), where the wonders of the human mind come to life. This cutting-edge method is rooted in the physiological theory that the brain's incredible workings, where neurons are constantly "firing," are intricately linked to an increase in blood flow within specific regions of the brain. Prepare to delve into the fascinating world of fMRI and unlock the secrets of the mind! Discover the fascinating world of MRI signs, where hidden clues reveal the subtle changes in blood flow. Uncover the secrets that lie within these enigmatic images and unlock a deeper understanding of the human body. Prepare to be amazed by the indirect information that awaits you. Discover the incredible insights that can be gleaned from this cutting-edge transmission. Researchers are able to infer the precise positioning and intensity of activity associated with various tasks, including the captivating act of reading individual words. All of this is made possible by the advanced technology of the scanner, providing invaluable data for analysis participants. Discover the fascinating world of research with data collected from diverse groups of individuals, providing valuable insights for scientific exploration. Please note that these studies are conducted solely for research purposes and not intended for diagnosing individuals with dyslexia.

Discover the Fascinating Brain Areas that Light Up When You're Reading!

Discover the fascinating origins of reading, a remarkable cultural invention that emerged as modern humans evolved. Unlike other cognitive processes, reading does not have a specific location within the mind that serves as a dedicated reading center. Explore the intricate complexities of this unique human ability. Discover the fascinating way our brains adapt and repurpose certain areas to facilitate reading. Rather than relying on pre-existing structures, the brain cleverly utilizes regions originally dedicated to tasks like spoken vocabulary and object identification (Dehaene & Cohen, 2007). Discover the fascinating world of reading, where multiple cognitive procedures come into play. Among these procedures, two have captured the attention of analysts:

Experience the power of grapheme-phoneme mapping, where a symphony of characters (graphemes) harmoniously blend with their corresponding sounds (phonemes), creating a mesmerizing process of decoding.

Discover the power of visible word form acknowledgement, a revolutionary technique that allows you to effortlessly map familiar words onto their mental representations. Experience the seamless integration of language and cognition like never before. Discover the incredible power of these methods that enable us to effortlessly pronounce words and unlock their profound meaning.

Discover the fascinating world of reading and its incredible impact on the human brain. Recent studies conducted on both adults and children have revealed a remarkable network of brain areas in the left hemisphere that support this essential skill. These areas include the occipito-temporal, temporo-parietal, and inferior frontal cortices. Dive into the science behind reading and unlock the secrets of the mind. Introducing the remarkable occipito-temporal cortex, home to the awe-inspiring "visible phrase form area". Experience the incredible synergy of the temporo-parietal and poor frontal cortices as they engage in the captivating world of phonological and semantic processing of words. Witness the remarkable involvement of the poor frontal cortex in the intricate formation of speech sounds. Prepare to be amazed by the intricate dance of these brain regions! Discover the groundbreaking research that has proven the transformative power of these areas in reshaping our understanding of human cognition. As demonstrated by Turkeltaub et al. (2003), these areas have the remarkable ability to adapt and evolve over time. Furthermore, individuals with dyslexia have been shown to experience significant modifications in these very same areas, as highlighted by Richlan et al. (2011). Prepare to be amazed by the incredible potential of these areas to revolutionize our understanding of the human brain.

Discover the fascinating insights that brain images have unveiled about the intricate framework of the brain in individuals with dyslexia.

Discover the fascinating link between dyslexia and the intricate framework of the mind through groundbreaking research. Pioneering scientists have uncovered compelling evidence by meticulously examining the anatomical structure of the brains of deceased adults who lived with dyslexia. Prepare to be amazed by the remarkable findings that shed light on this captivating connection. Experience the fascinating world of brain asymmetry in the left hemisphere temporal lobe, where the left-greater-than-right asymmetry is typically observed. However, in these remarkable brains, this asymmetry was not found, as revealed by Galaburda and Kemper in 1979. Additionally, the intriguing phenomenon of ectopias, which involves the displacement of brain cells to the very best of the brain, was also documented by Galaburda et al. in 1985. Prepare to be amazed by the wonders of neuroscience! Introducing the groundbreaking use of MRI technology, researchers embarked on a journey to unlock the secrets hidden within the intricate structures of the human brain. With unwavering determination, they delved into the minds of research volunteers, both those with and without dyslexia, capturing stunningly detailed structural images that would forever change the way we understand this enigmatic condition. Discover the cutting-edge imaging techniques that have unveiled a fascinating revelation: a reduction in the quantity of grey and white matter, along with a transformation in the integrity of white matter. These remarkable changes have been observed in the occipito-temporal and temporo-parietal areas of the left hemisphere. Discover how the intricate details of your email address are intricately influenced by your unique vocabulary and writing systems, as experts continue to delve into this fascinating subject.

Discover the Astonishing Insights Unveiled by Brain Images on Brain Function in Dyslexia!

Experience the groundbreaking world of early functional studies, where adults took center stage and pushed the boundaries of science with their daring use of cutting-edge invasive techniques and the mesmerizing allure of radioactive materials. Experience the groundbreaking advancements in brain mapping with the revolutionary invention of fMRI. Introducing the groundbreaking fMRI technology that ensures the utmost safety for both children and adults, without the need for any radioactive tracers. With its remarkable versatility, fMRI can be utilized on a regular basis, making it the perfect tool for conducting longitudinal studies on development and involvement. Introducing a groundbreaking tool in the study of dyslexia, fMRI made its debut in 1996 (Eden et al., 1996). Since then, it has become the go-to method for investigating the intricate workings of the brain when it comes to reading, including its various components such as phonology, orthography, and semantics. Discoveries from various countries have come together to reveal the remarkable findings of altered left-hemisphere regions (Richlan et al., 2011). These include the ventral occipito-temporal, temporo-parietal, and second-rate frontal cortices, along with their interconnected networks. Discover the undeniable truth: studies have unequivocally confirmed the universal presence of dyslexia across a multitude of diverse world dialects.

Discover the fascinating world of Genes, Brain Chemistry, and Brain Function.

Discover the fascinating world of dyslexia as we delve into the intricate web of hereditary variants. Uncover the ongoing investigations into the brain's response to these variants, both in humans and our furry friends, the mice. Prepare to be captivated by the latest research! Discover the fascinating world of research as experts delve into the intricate connection between genes associated with dyslexia and their potential impact on brain development and communication. Uncover the secrets hidden within specially bred pets and gain insights into the fascinating realm of neuroscience. Discover how these captivating investigations seamlessly align with groundbreaking studies in humans. Discover the fascinating world of brain anatomy and function! Recent studies by Darki et al. (2012) and Meda et al. (2008) have revealed intriguing variations in brain structure. But that's not all - Deal et al. (2012) and Pinel et al. (2012) have also uncovered remarkable differences in brain function. And here's the twist: these differences have been observed not only in individuals with dyslexia-associated genes, but even in those who possess exceptional reading abilities. Prepare to be amazed! Moreover, in addition to these meticulous investigations conducted at the anatomical, physiological, and molecular levels, researchers must strive to identify the precise chemical connection associated with dyslexia.

Introducing an incredible breakthrough: the power to visualize brain metabolites that play a crucial role in facilitating neuron communication. And how do we achieve this remarkable feat? Through the cutting-edge MRI-based technique known as spectroscopy.

Discover the fascinating world of metabolites and their intriguing connection to dyslexia. In a groundbreaking study by Pugh et al. (2014), it was revealed that individuals with dyslexia exhibit distinct variations in certain metabolites, such as choline. Uncover the secrets hidden within these metabolic differences and gain a deeper understanding of dyslexia like never before. Discover the ongoing exploration by experts as they delve into the intricate connections between these remarkable results. Their unwavering hope lies in the potential to uncover the very origins of dyslexia, paving the way for a deeper understanding of this complex condition. Discover the fascinating complexities of dyslexia research, where the intricate workings of the human brain hold the key to unraveling the mysteries behind reading difficulties. While it's true that not all reading issues can be attributed solely to differences in brain structure among individuals with dyslexia, it's important to consider other factors, such as the amount of reading one engages in. Explore the multifaceted nature of this captivating field and delve into the various factors that contribute to reading challenges.

Experience the transformative power of reading with our revolutionary program, "Adjustments in Reading, Changes in the Mind." Immerse yourself in a world of knowledge and personal growth as you embark on a journey that will expand your horizons and reshape your thinking. Discover the profound impact that reading can have on your mind and unlock the doors to new perspectives and insights. Join

Discover the fascinating world of brain imaging research, where groundbreaking studies have uncovered remarkable anatomical and functional changes in the minds of individuals as they master the art of reading (Turkeltaub et al., 2003). But that's not all - these remarkable findings extend to children and adults with dyslexia who have undergone effective reading education, revealing even more about the incredible potential of the human brain (Krafnick et al., 2011; Eden et al., 2004). Discover the fascinating insights that these studies provide into the intricate world of children with dyslexia. Uncover the remarkable advantages that reading instruction can bring to their brain-based variations. Witness the transformative benefits that these fortunate children experience, unlike their counterparts who do not receive such instruction. Unlock the power of neuroimaging data to predict the future of reading success for children, both with and without dyslexia.

Causes versus Consequences: Unveiling the Underlying Factors and Unraveling the Impact

Unlocking the secrets of the mind and reading is a crucial area of research. One intriguing question is whether the discoveries made could be the root cause or a result of dyslexia. Delving into this inquiry promises to shed light on the intricate relationship between the mind and the challenges of reading. Discover the astonishing impact of learning to read on the brain! Recent studies have revealed that the very same brain areas linked to dyslexia can undergo remarkable transformations when individuals acquire the skill of reading. Fascinating research conducted on adults who were once illiterate but have since learned to read has shed light on this incredible phenomenon (Carreiras et al., 2009). Discover the fascinating world of longitudinal studies in typical individuals, where groundbreaking research has uncovered remarkable anatomical changes that occur with each passing generation. These changes have been found to be closely linked to the process of development, as highlighted by the groundbreaking work of Giedd et al. (1999). Additionally, these studies have shed light on the incredible impact of language skills, with findings from Sowell et al. (2004) revealing a direct correlation between anatomical changes and the development of language proficiency. Furthermore, the research conducted by Lu et al. (2007) has shown that these changes in brain structure are intricately connected to improvements in phonological skills, providing further evidence of the remarkable plasticity of the human brain. Discover the fascinating world of brain-based distinctions that analysts are currently unraveling. These distinctions, observed even before children embark on their reading journey, shed light on the variations that arise due to dyslexia. Dive into the intriguing realm of reading differences and their impact on individuals with dyslexia. Discover the fascinating findings of experts who have uncovered modified brain anatomy (Raschle, et al., 2011) and function (Raschle, et al., 2012) in pre-reading children with a family background of dyslexia. Discover the exciting possibilities of future studies that utilize longitudinal designs, providing valuable insights into the timeline of adjustments and shedding light on the causes and consequences of anatomical and functional differences in dyslexia.

Discover the Fascinating World of Practical Brain Differences

Introducing the remarkable world of brain imaging! Discover the cutting-edge technique known as Functional Magnetic Resonance Imaging (fMRI). This noninvasive and relatively new method harnesses the power of a strong magnet to precisely detect blood flow, providing invaluable insights into neural activation. Prepare to be amazed by the wonders of fMRI! Introducing the revolutionary "practical" method! Imagine being able to perform tasks while in (or under) the magnet, unlocking the true potential of your working brain. Say goodbye to the limitations of a resting mind and embrace a whole new level of productivity.

Discover the fascinating world of dyslexia through cutting-edge imaging techniques. Numerous studies have unveiled intriguing patterns of mind activation, highlighting key differences between readers with and without dyslexia. These findings hold the potential to unlock crucial insights into this complex condition. Discover the fascinating world of individuals with RD and their brain activity. Experts, like Shaywitz et al. (1998), have uncovered a remarkable pattern of under-activation in areas where they may be weaker, and an intriguing over-activation in other areas. Dive into the research and uncover the secrets of the brain.

This type of functional imaging research has just been utilized with children. Discover the fascinating world of imaging children, where challenges abound and every detail matters. One of the key factors contributing to these challenges is the absolute reliance on the participant's unwavering stillness during the scanning process. Dive into the complexities and intricacies of this captivating field.

Introducing the most extensive and meticulously conducted study to date, showcasing the groundbreaking findings in children's research. Discover the groundbreaking research conducted by Shaywitz et al. (2002) on a group of 144 exceptionally talented right-handed children. This study explored the fascinating world of reading difficulties (RD) by comparing brain activation in children with and without RD. Through a series of captivating in- and out-of-magnet tasks, the researchers delved into the intricate processes involved in reading. They meticulously examined the ability to identify letter names or sounds, decode nonsensical words, and decipher the meaning of real words. Prepare to be amazed by the remarkable findings!

Experience the astonishing results as non-impaired

readers showcase unparalleled levels of activation, surpassing even the remarkable achievements of children with dyslexia.

Discover the groundbreaking findings of Shaywitz et al. (2002) as they unveil a fascinating insight into the world of child development. Their research reveals that children who possess the remarkable ability to decode sounds exhibit heightened activation in the crucial reading areas of the left hemisphere, while experiencing reduced activation in the right hemisphere, when compared to children with reading difficulties. This remarkable discovery sheds new light on the intricate workings of the young mind.

Discover the groundbreaking insight that experts have uncovered about children with RD. It has been suggested that these young learners experience a disruption in the trunk reading systems located in the left hemisphere of their brains. These systems are crucial for developing skilled and fluent reading abilities. However, fear not! These resourceful youngsters have found a way to compensate for this challenge. They tap into other, albeit less efficient, systems to continue their reading journey.

Discover the groundbreaking revelation that sheds light on the common phenomenon experienced by students with dyslexia. Despite their ability to achieve accuracy in reading, these students often struggle with slow and laborious reading of grade-level texts, lacking the essential element of fluency. (Torgesen, Rashotte, & Alexander, 2001)

Discover the fascinating world of dyslexia, where the mind of an individual takes on a unique distribution of metabolic activation. Unlike those without reading difficulties, the brain of someone with dyslexia showcases a distinct pattern when tackling vocabulary tasks. Explore the intricacies of this extraordinary condition today! Discover the incredible impact of the left hemisphere back brain systems on reading and unlock their full potential.

Discover the fascinating world of dyslexia, where individuals often exhibit heightened activation in the reduced frontal regions of the mind. Discover the fascinating phenomenon where neural systems in frontal areas rise to the occasion, compensating for disruptions in the posterior area. As revealed by Shaywitz et al. (2003), this leads to the ultimate result. Discover the intriguing potential of utilizing brain imaging as a cutting-edge diagnostic tool to identify college students with reading disabilities. This captivating information is sure to leave teachers questioning the possibilities.

Discover the power of inclusivity by revealing the individuals who may face challenges with reading.

Discover the untapped potential that awaits. The journey to greatness begins now. Imagine the captivating scene of placing a child we deeply care for in an fMRI machine, swiftly and accurately identifying their condition. However, it's worth noting that research on this groundbreaking technology is still relatively limited.

Discover the multitude of reasons why the current feasibility of utilizing imaging methods in clinical or school-based settings to identify children with dyslexia is limited. Introducing the unparalleled expense of fMRI machines, personal computers, and the indispensable program required to operate them. Discover the hidden expenses that may arise when it comes to personnel required to execute and analyze the results.

Introducing the groundbreaking technology designed to revolutionize diagnosis accuracy for individuals. Experience the future of precision with this cutting-edge diagnostic tool. Introducing the latest breakthrough in communication technology - email details! With their unparalleled reliability, email details are the go-to solution for reporting information for sets of participants. However, it's important to note that they may not be as effective for individuals within each group (Richards, 2001; Shaywitz et al., 2002). Experience the power of email details today!

Discover the remarkable potential of imaging methods for diagnosing individual children by minimizing the occurrence of false negatives and false positives. By accurately identifying children with problems and distinguishing those who are truly average, we can revolutionize the way we diagnose and support our young ones.

Chapter 4

Discover the Telltale Signs of Dyslexia

Discovering indicators of dyslexia in your child before they start school can be challenging. However, there are several early clues that may suggest a potential problem. Discover the invaluable role of your child's teacher as the first line of defense in identifying potential issues as your little one embarks on their educational journey. Discover the varying degrees of severity, as this common issue often reveals itself when a young child embarks on the exciting journey of learning to read.

Experience the magic of the early morning with our exclusive "Before School" program. Start your day off right with a range of activities designed to energize and inspire.

Discover the telltale signs that could indicate a young child's susceptibility to dyslexia.

- One such sign is late talking.

- Discover the art of expanding your vocabulary at a

leisurely pace.

Introducing a revolutionary solution for those struggling with word formation! Say goodbye to the frustration of reversing sounds in words or mixing up words that sound alike. Our innovative approach will help you conquer these challenges with ease. Experience the power of clear and accurate word formation like never before!

Introducing our revolutionary solution for those struggling with memory and word recall! Say goodbye to the frustration of forgetting words, digits, and even colors. Our cutting-edge technology is here to help you effortlessly remember and name with ease. Experience the power of enhanced memory today!

Discover the joy of nursery rhymes and rhyming games with ease!

Discover the Excitement of School Age!

Discover the telltale signs of dyslexia that may become more apparent once your child enters college:

Discover the captivating world of reading, where every

page holds the key to imagination and knowledge. Unlock the power of words and embark on a literary journey that will transport you to new horizons. Explore the vast realm of literature and embrace the joy of reading, transcending age and expectations.

Introducing a revolutionary solution for those struggling with auditory comprehension and control. Say goodbye to the frustration of not being able to fully understand and process what you hear. Our cutting-edge technology is here to empower you and transform your listening experience. Experience the difference today!

Struggling to find the perfect phrase or craft well-thought-out answers to questions?

Introducing the revolutionary solution for those who struggle with remembering a group of things.

Discover a whole new level of visual and auditory perception with our cutting-edge technology. Say goodbye to the struggle of recognizing similarities and differences in characters and words. Experience a world of clarity and precision like never before.

Discover the frustration of struggling to articulate the pronunciation of a brand new word.

Struggling with spelling? We've got you covered!

Discover the art of immersing yourself in the world of words and ideas, as you spend an extraordinary amount of time effortlessly conquering tasks that require the delicate balance of reading and writing.

Discover the art of indulging in activities that don't require reading.

Discover the Telltale Signs of Teenagers and Adults.

Discover how dyslexia symptoms can persist and impact teenagers and adults, just as they do in children. Discover the telltale signs of dyslexia in teenagers and adults:

Experience the challenge of reading, even when it comes to reading aloud.

Experience the ease and efficiency of reading and writing like never before with our innovative solution. Say goodbye to sluggishness and laboriousness, and say hello to a seamless and effortless experience.

Introducing: The Ultimate Solution for Spelling Woes!

Discover the art of avoiding activities that require reading.

Introducing: The Ultimate Language Mastery Solution! Say goodbye to mispronounced titles and forgotten words with our revolutionary language tool. Never again will you stumble over words or struggle to retrieve the right vocabulary. Experience seamless communication and impress everyone with your flawless pronunciation. *Unlock the power of language mastery today!*

Discover the secret to effortlessly unraveling the mysteries of jokes and expressions that hide their true meaning within the confines of mere words. Say goodbye to the confusion of idioms and embrace a world of linguistic clarity.

Discover the joy of immersing yourself in tasks that involve reading or writing, and savor the extra time you spend on them.

Struggling to condense and capture the essence of an account? Look no further! Our expert summarization services are here to save the day. Say goodbye to the frustration of trying to distill complex information into a concise and compelling summary. Let us handle the heavy lifting and deliver a

- Having trouble mastering the beautiful language of Spanish?

- Struggling to remember things?

- Struggling with math? Let us help you overcome the difficulty of solving mathematics problems.

Discover the Perfect Time to Consult a Doctor

Discover the fascinating journey of learning to read. While many children embark on this adventure in kindergarten or 1st grade, there are some exceptional individuals who face unique challenges. Children with dyslexia, for instance, may find it difficult to grasp the fundamental principles of reading during this crucial period. Discover the power of consulting with a highly skilled medical doctor if your child's reading level falls below the expected standards of their generation. Don't hesitate to seek professional advice if you notice any additional telltale signs of dyslexia. Your child's future success may depend on it.

Discover the detrimental effects of undiagnosed and untreated dyslexia, as the struggle with reading persists from childhood well into adulthood.

Discover the Hidden Risks of Dyslexia

Discover the key risk factors associated with dyslexia, a condition that affects millions of individuals worldwide. One of the primary risk factors is having a family background with dyslexia or other learning disabilities. Uncover the fascinating insights into this complex condition and its genetic links.

Experience the potential risks of premature delivery or low birth weight.

Discover the potential risks that can impact your precious bundle of joy during pregnancy. From exposure to smoking, drugs, alcohol consumption, to harmful contaminants, learn how these factors can potentially alter the delicate development of your baby's brain.

Discover the fascinating world of person distinctions in the components of the mind that unlock the power of reading.

Introducing: Complications.

Discover the multitude of challenges that can arise from dyslexia, such as:

Discover the solution to your learning challenges: Unlock the potential of every child with dyslexia by recognizing that reading is not just a skill, but an art that forms the foundation of countless other subjects. Unfortunately, this unique learning challenge can put them at a disadvantage in most classes, making it difficult for them to keep up with their peers. Let's empower these children to overcome their obstacles and thrive.

Introducing dyslexia, a condition that, if left untreated, can lead to a range of social problems. From low self-esteem to behavioral issues, stress to aggression, and even withdrawal from friends, parents, and instructors. Don't let dyslexia hold you back. Take action today.

Discover the challenges we face as adults: Unlock the full potential of your child's growth by eliminating the barriers of understanding and comprehension. Don't let these shortcomings hold them back from reaching new heights! Experience the transformative power of this incredible opportunity, unlocking a world of long-term educational, interpersonal, and economic benefits.

Introducing the all-new and improved "•"! This revolutionary product is here to change the game. Get ready to experience Discover the fascinating connection between dyslexia and attention-deficit/hyperactivity disorder (ADHD) in children. It's a two-way street, as children with dyslexia are at an increased risk of developing ADHD, and vice versa. Discover the powerful impact of ADHD on attention, hyperactivity, and impulsive behavior. Uncover how these challenges can intensify the struggle of managing dyslexia.

Chapter 5

Discover the 20 telltale signs of dyslexia!

Discover the early signs of a learning impairment that can emerge during the crucial preschool years. Discover the unique world of dyslexia, where each case is as extraordinary as the individual themselves. Despite the individuality, there are several shared characteristics and behaviors that unite those with dyslexia. Introducing our comprehensive compilation of the top twenty most prevalent dyslexia symptoms. This invaluable resource will empower you to effortlessly identify whether your child is at risk level. Don't miss out on this essential tool!

Discover the truth: symptoms of dyslexia are not causes, but rather indicators of this unique condition. Introducing a collection of ideas, presented in a captivating manner, without any specific sequence:

- The Ultimate Solution for Reading Challenges!

- Struggling with spelling words in your written work? Look no further!

- Introducing the solution to your low self-confidence or behavioral problems.

- Introducing the remarkable ability to effortlessly reverse letters and/or quantities with ease. Say goodbye to transposing errors forever!

- Experience flawless pronunciation.

- Experience the power of silence and simplicity with our revolutionary reading and writing technique. Say goodbye to unnecessary noise and words as you immerse yourself in a world of focused and efficient communication.

- Introducing the ultimate solution for those pesky headaches.

- Experience the challenge of reading aloud like never before.

- Introducing: The Ultimate Solution for Directional Dilemmas!

- Introducing the revolutionary solution to all your

writing woes - the impeccable writing tools! Say goodbye to those pesky issues with pencils or pens and experience a whole new level of writing perfection.

- Introducing: The Solution to Your Sequenced Instruction Struggles!

- Introducing a revolutionary approach to reading: no more guessing, missing, or updating words! Say goodbye to the struggle of sounding out words and embrace a new way of reading with ease.

- Discover a unique combination of exceptional dental expertise and a humble reading ability.

- Experience the magic of letters that come to life on the page, dancing and twirling with a mesmerizing grace. Witness the captivating phenomenon of letters that may seem blurry or delightfully out of place, adding an element of intrigue to your reading experience.

- Struggling with business and time management?

We've got you covered!

- Introducing the revolutionary solution to the problem of failing to differentiate talk sounds.

- Experience the challenge of effortlessly repeating phrases or sentences.

- Feeling crushed by disappointing grades?

- Introducing a revolutionary solution: Say goodbye to flash bank cards and memorization! Our cutting-edge technology will transform the way you handle your finances.

- Discover the transformative power of reading below your peers' quality level.

Unleash the Power of Dyslexia

Experience the awe-inspiring beauty of the grand panorama.

Discover the unique perspective of individuals with

dyslexia, who possess a remarkable ability to see the bigger picture. Experience the enchantment of rediscovering the beauty of the trees, while simultaneously gaining a newfound appreciation for the majestic forest that surrounds them.

Discover the fascinating perspective of individuals with dyslexia. It's like they have a wide-angle contact lens that allows them to see the world in a unique way. On the other hand, some individuals use a telephoto lens, which helps them uncover different types of fine details. Both approaches have their strengths and reveal a whole new level of understanding. Introducing Matthew H. Schneps, the brilliant mind behind his groundbreaking work at Harvard University.

Discovering the extraordinary outlier Unleashing the power of dyslexic individuals who excel in global visual processing and the identification of improbable figures. Discover the fascinating world of dyslexic scientist Christopher Tonkin, whose extraordinary degree of sensitivity to "things out of place" will leave you in awe. Introducing the remarkable researchers who possess the extraordinary ability to make sense of vast amounts of visual data and flawlessly identify enigmatic black hole anomalies.

Discover the remarkable rise of individuals with dyslexia in the captivating realm of neuro-scientific astrophysics. Prepare to be amazed by the groundbreaking research conducted at the prestigious Harvard-Smithsonian Centre for Astrophysics. Discover the fascinating findings that confirm individuals with dyslexia possess a remarkable ability to discern and commit intricate visuals to memory.

Experience the power of enhanced pattern recognition.

Discover the remarkable abilities of individuals with dyslexia as they effortlessly navigate the intricate world of connecting elements to form harmonious organic systems. Witness their unique talent for recognizing patterns and uncovering striking similarities among a multitude of objects. Prepare to be amazed by their extraordinary perception and astute observations. Experience the remarkable benefits that are especially valuable in fields such as technology and mathematics, where visual representations are essential.

Discover the incredible journey of self-discovery as I unlocked the hidden power of my mind, harnessing the extraordinary gift of imagination, all while coming to terms with my dyslexia. Welcome to my extraordinary abode, a realm adorned with mesmerizing patterns and captivating images. Within these walls, I possess the remarkable ability to perceive the unseen, unveiling a world that remains hidden to others. Unlock the power of dyslexia and unleash your ability to uncover hidden patterns.

Discover the power of working around dyslexia and harnessing its potential to work for you. While it may never completely disappear, you can overcome its challenges and create a path to success. Discover the undeniable importance of dyslexia, as it holds the key to unlocking your unique set of talents and gifts. Without it, your other remarkable abilities would simply fade away into oblivion.

Discover the power of sound spatial knowledge

Unlock the hidden potential of individuals with dyslexia as they showcase their remarkable ability to effortlessly manipulate 3D objects within the depths of their brilliant minds. Discover the fascinating truth that lies behind the genius of many of the world's most renowned architects and fashion designers - they possess the remarkable gift of dyslexia.

Unlocking the Power of Dyslexia

Discover the power of resilience. Despite facing adversity, I have been called stupid. Discover the incredible challenge I faced: the inability to read and the struggle to memorize my assignment work. Are you tired of always being at the bottom of the class? It's time to make a change and rise to the top! Say goodbye to being left behind and hello to success. Let's transform your academic journey together! Experience the depths of despair like never before. Introducing Richard Rogers - a name that resonates with excellence and innovation. With a remarkable track record in his field, Richard Rogers is a true visionary. His expertise

"Unlock your true potential at college! Despite facing challenges like dyslexia, I persevered and overcame the odds. Don't let anyone label you as 'stupid' - rise above and prove them wrong!" Experience the thrill of reading like never before! Experience the power of unwavering focus as you effortlessly navigate from left to right on our website. No more distractions, no more wandering vision. Concentrate with ease and achieve the ideal browsing experience you've always desired. Experience the timeless elegance of Tommy Hilfiger.

Unlock the Power of Visual Thinking

Unlock the extraordinary power of the mind with dyslexia. Experience a unique way of thinking, where vibrant pictures replace ordinary words. Embrace the visual world of dyslexia and discover a whole new dimension of thought. Discover the groundbreaking research conducted at the prestigious University of California, revealing a remarkable breakthrough for children with dyslexia. This cutting-edge study has demonstrated a significant enhancement in the storage of picture recognition, offering new hope and possibilities for these young minds.

Experience the captivating world of the renowned nineteenth-century French sculptor, Auguste Rodin. With an unwavering passion for art, Rodin would spend his days immersed in the masterpieces adorning museum walls, only to continue his artistic journey by night, meticulously recreating these paintings from the depths of storage. Witness the extraordinary talent and dedication of this visionary artist as he breathes life into his own interpretations of these timeless works of art. Unlocking the power of words proved to be a challenge for him. His dyslexia, a unique design of his mind, prevented him from effortlessly reading or writing by the tender age of fourteen. However, like a blossoming flower, his reading skills emerged gracefully, albeit at a slightly delayed pace.

Experience the power of enhanced peripheral vision

Discover the remarkable advantage of individuals with dyslexia - their exceptional peripheral eyesight. With this unique ability, they effortlessly absorb the entirety of a scene, capturing every detail in a single glance. Discover the hidden advantage of dyslexia: it enhances your ability to perceive external boundaries, even if articulating it in precise terms may pose a challenge.

Unleash Your Inner Business Genius!

Discover the astonishing fact that one in three American companies are affected by dyslexia.

Discover the remarkable stories of dyslexic visionaries such as Thomas Edison, Henry Ford, Steve Jobs, and Charles Schwab. These extraordinary individuals defied the odds and achieved greatness, proving that dyslexia is no barrier to success. Unlock the true potential of your business with the power of strategic thinking and creative innovation. Experience tangible business benefits like never before.

Discover the power of your unique perspective, setting

you apart from your classmates. Discover the power of unwavering focus as you embark on the journey of building your very own company and bringing your vision to life. Discover the incredible impact of my dyslexia on revolutionizing our customer communication. Introducing the one and only Richard Branson!

Unleash your imagination with our highly creative solutions.

Discover the fascinating world of dyslexia, where creativity knows no bounds. Join the ranks of iconic stars like Johnny Depp, Keira Knightley, and Orlando Bloom, who have defied all odds to become true visionaries.

"Discover the secret of super developers who effortlessly overcome dyslexia and excel in their field. Uncover the essential aspect they employ to keep their experience free from any hindrances. Join the ranks of these exceptional individuals and unlock your true potential." Introducing Soren Petersen, the brilliant mind behind groundbreaking design research. With a Ph.D. to his name, Soren is a true expert in his field. Prepare to be amazed by his innovative ideas and unparalleled expertise.

Introducing Pablo Picasso: The Master Designer

Discover the extraordinary genius of Picasso, a true master of art, who was once described by his educators as having a unique ability to challenge the traditional orientation of characters. Experience the genius of Picasso as he fearlessly brings his subjects to life, painting them with a unique perspective that defies convention. With a bold disregard for traditional norms, Picasso's vibrant strokes capture the essence of his subjects, whether they are presented in a seemingly random sequence, reversed, or even in their raw, unfiltered form. Witness the extraordinary artistry of Picasso as he fearlessly embraces the unconventional, creating masterpieces that challenge the boundaries of beauty. Experience the awe-inspiring mastery of his brushstrokes, as his paintings effortlessly showcase the boundless depths of his creative genius. It is said that his unparalleled talent may have stemmed from a unique perspective, a beautiful quirk that allowed him to transcend the limitations of written language.

Unleash your creativity with out-of-the-box thinking - the key to effective problem solving!

Discover the fascinating world of individuals with dyslexia, renowned for their remarkable ability to uncover groundbreaking solutions through unconventional thinking.

Discover the power of an innovative problem-solving technique that transcends traditional methods and embraces the art of daydreaming. Experience the unique perspective of dyslexics as they effortlessly navigate the world through their windows. Witness their brain effortlessly unravel complex problems, effortlessly assembling connections with natural ease and simplicity.

Acknowledgements

Behold the magnificent triumph of this extraordinary book, a testament to the divine intervention of God Almighty and the unwavering love and support of my cherished Family, devoted Fans, avid Readers, loyal Customers, and dear Friends. Their ceaseless encouragement has paved the way for this resounding success.

www.ingramcontent.com/pod-product-compliance
Lightning Source LLC
Chambersburg PA
CBHW031906200326
41597CB00012B/544